20 PRACTICAL LIFESTYLE AND VALUABLE TIPS TO COPE AFTER BABY ARRIVED

Experience of parenthood.

By

Dr TIMOTHY KESSINGTON

approval from the publisher or creator.

TABLE OF CONTENTS

ABOUT THE AUTHOR

INTRODUCTION.

TABLE OF CONTENTS

ABOUT THE AUTHOR

Dr. TIMOTHY KESSINGTON is a licensed psychologist in the state of texas. he is a certified counselor on marriage and relationship/mental health. He is passionate to the core to see people in relationships happy and couples achieve the best out of every relationship.

INTRODUCTION

While being a parent is a wonderful experience, there are many new difficulties involved. Your life will significantly alter when the baby is born, and navigating this new phase might be difficult. Yet, you can adapt to your new work and make the transition much easier with the appropriate practical lifestyle and helpful advice. In this article, we'll go over twenty crucial suggestions for handling postpartum life.

CHAPTER 1

ALL YOUR TIME IS BABY TIME.

Congratulations! The timetable of your child is now your own. Babies sleep for up to 18 hours per day. It is divided into manageable portions, and in between, there is feeding, diaper-changing, and a lot of hugging and cooing.

Tip: Baby naps become longer and more regular after the first frantic weeks. Your ability to manage your time will improve.

CHAPTER 2

SLEEP ENOUGH.

The lack of sleep is among the most difficult elements of raising a baby. It is important to emphasize rest if you want to manage after the baby is born. Whenever possible, try to snooze whenever the infant does, even if it's only for a little nap. Make sure the space where you sleep is peaceful and cozy.

Advice; If you can, ask a spouse or member of your family to monitor the infant while you get some rest.

CHAPTER 3

YOU'VE JOINED A WORLDWIDE CLUB.

It is known as parenting. All of a sudden, you have plenty of pals. Strangers give you a grin. Moms invite you to join them for a play date at church or the temple. Your employer is curious about the outcome of the baby's healthcare appointment. Enjoin the pleasant company!

Advice: You'll create a unique parenting approach that works for your family.

CHAPTER 4

YOUR RELATIONSHIP CHANGES.

With one additional person to communicate with, "we" will have less time. You could get so busy that you forget to communicate because the dynamics of your relationship are different. If one of you looks after the infant most of the time, the other person could feel neglected.

Tip: Schedule time exclusively for the two of you. Set up a date and discuss your life's current events.

CHAPTER 5

Develop a routine

Infants thrive on routine, so creating one may make you feel more in control and less stressed out. Establish a flexible schedule that incorporates playtime, naptime, and feeding times.

Tip: If you follow this plan as closely as you can, your baby will become used to it soon, making your days easier.

CHAPTER 6

A NEW NIGHT-TIME SCHEDULE.

It is real. Seldom does having a new baby equate to restful sleep. While this should only last a short while, you may alternate getting up with your spouse while your infant sleeps through the night.

Tip: Don't attempt to do duties while the baby is sleeping throughout the day. Repose on the ground.

CHAPTER 7

You will get a ton of visitors

Family and friends will undoubtedly want to meet the newborn. (And they'll offer tales of raising their children as well as suggestions for rearing yours.) Before letting anybody touch the baby, make sure none of the visitors are contagious and have them wash their hands.

Tip: Do you feel overburdened or worn out? Saying "Let's make it another time" is acceptable. Most people will understand.

CHAPTER 8

Take good maintenance of yourself.

It's easy to forget about your personal needs when concentrating only on the kid. Self-care, however, is crucial for coping after the baby is born. Whenever you can, set aside some time for yourself, even if it's only for a little while. Take a soothing bath, read a book, or stretch out gently. Consume balanced meals, drink plenty of water, and make an effort to exercise whenever you can.

TIP: Keep in mind that caring for yourself is not selfish; it is vital for both your physical and emotional well-being.

CHAPTER 9

YOUR FACE CAN DO WEIRD THINGS.

Infants pick up new skills through observing and interacting with their surroundings. You'll find yourself making silly faces to cheer up your infant. Over the first few weeks, you'll notice that your child is studying before finally copying your goofy expressions.

Tip: To get their attention, give a smile, stick out your tongue, or make a silly noise.

CHAPTER 10

YOU NEED HELP.

While they are adorable, babies need a lot of care. Try not to embark on it by yourself. Each day, while the other is caring for the infant, you should both have time to yourselves. Read a book, take a stroll, take a bath, or watch a favorite TV program.

Tip: Being a single parent? Ask a friend or family member to help out. A break allows you to rejuvenate.

CHAPTER 11

.BABIES REQUIRE CONVERSATION.

Talking to your infant fosters both your relationship and their learning. And such things happen more often the more you communicate. Just keep this in mind. To learn to speak, your infant needs to hear actual words.

Advice: First, make the noises that your baby makes, such as "ba-ba" or "goo-goo," then wait for them to produce another sound before repeating it back. This aids in their acquisition of conversational give and take.

CHAPTER 12

GUILT IS NATURAL.

You promised yourself that you would be a great parent. Nonetheless, you can sometimes yearn for your former life and then feel terrible for not savoring every moment of motherhood. It's not just you! It seems to make sense to need a break from the infant.

Tip: Call a buddy after he is secure in the crib. Praise yourself for all the things that are going well and give yourself a break.

Chapter 13:

SEEK ASSISTANCE.

Asking for assistance is a show of strength, not weakness. Asking for help from family, friends, or a postpartum doula is nothing to be ashamed of. They may assist with chores like cooking, cleaning, or babysitting so you can take a much-needed break.

TIP: At this trying time, accepting aid may also make you feel less overwhelmed and more supported.

CHAPTER 14

CHILDREN'S BOOKS ARE LITERATURE.

If you weren't familiar with children's literature before, you will be after reading this. Several books are created with parents and kids in mind. They both amuse and instruct. It's never too early to begin reading to your baby since they adore it.

Advice: Reading aloud to your child can help them recognize words later on.

CHAPTER 15

YOU WILL MAKE MISTAKES.

Maybe there are ideal parents in a perfect world. Do what works is the common guideline in the actual world. You should agree if your kid uses a pacifier to fall asleep even if she is too old for one. Give yourself a break; it won't harm her.

Advice: See your doctor if you're unsure.

CHAPTER 16

YOU BECOME A JUDGE.

Your function as a mediator changes as your kid matures. There will be limits to set, sibling conflicts to resolve, and timeouts to keep an eye on. While it's not always simple to enforce discipline, it's an essential element of the work. Also, it's good for your youngsters.

Tip: Make aside time to spend with each child separately so they each feel important and get your full attention.

CHAPTER 17

YOU GET A BATHROOM BUDDY

You won't begin potty training your new baby for a few years. You or your partner should be prepared for a crowd when you do. Parent modeling is one approach to educating children about the need of using the restroom.

Advice: Children not only pick up on words but also on deeds.

CHAPTER 18

BABY LOVE IS REAL

For some parents, it happens right away; for others, it could take some time. One day, when you gaze at your kid, you'll experience a level of feeling you've never felt. It might be a wonderful surprise to realize just how limitless unconditional love is.

TIP: For a connection that will last a lifetime, enjoy it and build on it.

CHAPTER 19

CONNECT WITH OTHER PARENTS

Parenthood may be lonely, particularly if it's your first time. Making friends with other parents might make you feel less alone and provide you access to an invaluable support network. Attend parenting courses nearby, join a local parent group online, or do both.

TIP: It might be quite helpful to share your experiences with those who can relate to what you're going through.

CHAPTER 20

YOUR CHILD IS AN INVESTMENT.

Around $225,000 is typically spent by middle-class families over a child's first 18 years of life. Only to provide for basic needs like food, housing, and other things. Things like increases in health insurance premiums and college are excluded.

TIP: For maximum preparedness, start your financial preparation right now.

CONCLUSION

It might be difficult to cope when the baby is born, but with his realistic lifestyle and helpful advice, you can go through this new chapter more smoothly. Keep in mind that parenting is a journey filled with ups and downs and prioritize relaxation, build a routine, take care of yourself, seek support, and connect with other practical and lifestyle-type routes. You'll find your rhythm and appreciate this amazing experience with some time and patience.